Tantric Massage:

The Ultimate Beginners Guide to Tantric Massage Techniques

Table of Contents

Introduction

Tantric massages are massages that emphasize on the sexual energies of a person to create a pleasurable and relaxing state of mind. While many people believe Tantric massages are purely sexual, this is not actually true. Although the massage does use sexual energy to stimulate pleasure, the purpose is not to have intercourse but rather to create an overall sense of relaxation and calmness, as well as help people connect more intimately with their own bodies.

The common belief is that Tantric massages are primarily for females, but they are actually easy to accomplish for males as well. Everyone can benefit from the wonders of Tantric massages. This guide will show you exactly how you can create a sensual and effective Tantric massage for both women and men.

Throughout this book, you will learn some of the best techniques, skills, and extras you can accomplish in order to create an exceptional experience for your massage recipient. If you are ready to get started, read on!

Chapter 1
Tantra

While many people have a vague idea of what Tantra means, most are blissfully unaware of its true definition. Some believe it is purely based on sex, and others are entirely void of any idea as to what the term means. Tantra is a term used to describe the kind of energy that is used when completing tantric massages.

Is Tantra Sexual?

While Tantra does cover sexuality, it goes far beyond that as well. It is less about sex and more about lovemaking, as well as spirituality. While Tantric massages are sexual in nature and, when done in certain ways, can stimulate the sexual organs, their primary purpose is not to stimulate sex. Rather, it is to connect one closer with their physical being and draw them down a spiritual experience. It is intended to help individuals achieve enlightenment. Tantra itself covers various styles of yoga, dance, astrology, geometry, and several other things that are generally regarded as spiritually rooted.

One part of the Tantric path is lovemaking, which is where the connection to sex comes into play. It encourages people to look at sex as something deeper than simply two bodies physically stimulating one another. Rather, you view sex as a spiritual opportunity to connect with yourself and another individual on a deeper level. Tantra allows you to connect to your femininity if you are a female, or your masculinity if you are a male. It allows women to be women, and men to be men.

How to Learn Tantra

There are many opportunities for you to learn Tantra. While some people like to attend workshops and other group-like settings to learn about it, others would prefer to keep private matters private and learn through a book. This book is entirely designed to teach you exactly how you can use Tantra to stimulate your sex life and enhance the depth of your lovemaking experiences.

Chapter 2
Tantric Therapy

Tantric therapy is the art of using the Tantra lifestyle strategies to experience their sexuality in a unique way. It combines sexuality, massage therapy, and stimulation to create a sensual and spiritual experience for the recipient. There are various benefits of tantric therapy, with these benefits being unique to men and women. As such, we are going to explore each side independently so that you can develop a greater understanding of how tantric therapy can be a benefit to both you and your partner.

For Women

Tantric massage for women is a highly sexual experience that allows women to explore their sexuality. For women, there are actually 7 different types of orgasms, and all women can experience female ejaculation. Most women experience between 1-4 types of orgasms and very few experience female ejaculations through sex alone. By engaging in tantric massage a woman can experience each of these unique orgasm types as well as female ejaculation.

It may surprise you, but many women have not even experienced one type of orgasm in their life. Alternatively, they may struggle to orgasm from sex alone and therefore have never experienced an orgasm with their partner. Up to 30% of women have never experienced an orgasm, and approximately 40% of those who have experienced orgasms have only ever had a clitoris orgasm. This means that there is a lot of pleasurable experiences being neglected because women are unaware of the fact that they can achieve alternative orgasm styles, and may not know how to. They may begin to believe there is something wrong with them or that they simply are not capable of experiencing orgasms, but this is false. Every woman can experience 7 different orgasms, and every woman can experience female ejaculation. Tantric massage can enable women who have never had all of these experiences to have them for the first time.

Another time when Tantric massages can be beneficial for women is with women who have experienced emotional or physical trauma in their lifetime. These women may have been raped or sexually abused in some way and so they feel a lot of guilt, shame, or general discomfort about sex. When Tantric massages are used, women can learn to relax and enjoy sex once again without the emotional attachments and struggles that can arise during the act itself. Tantric massages of the yoni (vagina) can help with general vaginal health, as well.

For Men

While Tantric massages for women appear to be the most popular Tantric massages, there are variations available for men as well. These massages can have exceptionally valuable benefits to males, just like Yoni massages can have wonderful benefits for females.

It is not a surprise that men and women share differences in sexuality, including the fact that men are typically turned on the moment they touch a woman in bed whereas women can take some time to warm up. For men, Tantric massages can teach them to last longer, to be turned on by physical stimulation instead of mental or visual stimulation (such as porn), and to experience Tantra overall. Tantric massages can actually teach men to become multi-orgasmic so that they can last significantly longer and gain various climaxes from a single sexual encounter.

Most men experience an orgasm that provides about 3-5 seconds of explosive pleasure, and then they are exhausted and no longer want to have sex with their partner. Something incredible to learn is that men can orgasm without ejaculating, and Tantric massages can teach them exactly how to accomplish that. As a result, they can orgasm multiple times during sex without ever climaxing and, as a result, they can have a significantly more enjoyable sex life with their partner.

As with women, men who have experienced sexual abuse or trauma in their past can also be benefited from Tantric massages. It teaches them to open up and feel more comfortable with their sexuality and with intimacy itself. This allows them to have a more satisfying and enjoyable sex life overall, which means that both them and their partner can enjoy a closer sense of intimacy with each other that may not have been an option prior to the Tantric massages.

Are the Results Always the Same?

As with anything, the results will not always be the same from person to person. Some may have a wonderful experience with Tantric massages and open right up to the experience, whereas others may feel uncomfortable or not gain any benefits or pleasure from the experience. There are a few factors that contribute to how you will respond to your own massage experience. The primary factor is how open a person is (or isn't) to the experience. Someone who is open to the Tantric massage and willing to give it an honest shot is going to gain infinitely higher benefit rates than someone who is not open to it and is doing it because they feel pressured to or for some other reason. You should never feel pressured to try Tantric massages, as this pressure can actually destroy the purpose and benefit of the massage and ruin your experience overall. You should always experience Tantra because you *want* to.

The next common thing that matters is the quality of the massage the person experienced. When someone is just learning to give massages and testing out their abilities, they may not be able to provide the same value and benefit as someone who has been doing it for a long time. That is not to say that the beginner should not be given the opportunity to help, just to say that it may take slightly longer for the full benefits to be acquired due to their less experienced capabilities and skills.

Do You Need a Professional Massage?

Many people prefer to go to a professional Tantric massage therapist because these individuals have graduated from a course that teaches them exactly how to accomplish the massage properly. You can certainly choose a professional if you are interested in getting your massage done from someone who has experience and has been professionally trained in Tantra. However, there is nothing that requires you to go to a professional if you want to have a Tantric massage.

Several couples have discovered ways to self-teach Tantric massage methods so that they can perform these massages on one another. Doing this can develop the intimacy in your personal relationship and can also lead to a more romantic sexual relationship between you and your partner. This book will teach you exactly how you can perform Tantric massages on each other so that you can both gain the benefits of Tantra together.

Chapter 3
Tantric Massage for Women

As you learned in the previous chapter, there are many valuable benefits that can be gained by receiving a tantric massage if you are a woman. It can allow you to experience each of the seven different types of orgasms that are available to women. It can also help relieve past traumas from abuse or other sexual situations that were not comfortable to you.

You can perform Tantric massages on yourself, or you can have your trusted partner perform them on you if you so desire. For the purpose of simplicity, the following tutorial will be written as though you are practicing the massage on yourself. Your partner can simply improvise and take over if you would like to have the massage done by him or her.

How to Start

Before you get into the massage itself, you want to warm up for the experience. You want to start by opening your mind and your heart and freeing yourself of any judgment you may be experiencing. You should not judge yourself, your intentions, your body, or otherwise.

Have yourself lie down on your back in a position that is extremely comfortable for you. Place a pillow under your hips, prop your knees up, and put your feet firmly on the ground, bed, or whatever surface you are lying on. Ideally, you want to have your favorite massage oil handy for this experience. You want to stimulate as many of your senses as possible, and the massage oil will help you stimulate your physical body as well as your sense of smell.

Whenever you are completing a Tantra practice, you want to connect to your breath. This is important as it helps you connect to your body in a more holistic way which will lend itself to the overall experience. For this tutorial, you want to use a breath known as the "Bliss Breath". To do the Bliss Breath, you want to constrict the back of your throat and inhale so that you hear a whispering sound. Then, you can exhale and release the sound again. You want to continue doing this as you take deep, slow, and audible breaths.

When you breathe this way, your body becomes grounded and you are not stuck in your head during the experience. It helps you spread the orgasmic pleasure throughout your entire body which will help you have a full body orgasm. If you get stuck in your head, you risk having an orgasm that is restricted to your clitoris. While this is fine, it is not the ultimate goal with a Tantric massage. Having deep, consistent breathing can help you move the energy around and beyond your yoni.

During sexual intercourse, clitoris foreplay is often favored as it is a quick and sure-fire way to get a woman warmed up. For the Tantric massage, you want to avoid warming up this way and use other parts of the body to warm up instead. There are several areas on the female body with nerve endings that can stimulate pleasure, the goal is to simply find them and work with them.

Many areas that are often overlooked include the belly, the ribcage, space between your breasts, and your lower abdomen. As you massage these areas, your body will begin to respond to the sensation. When it begins responding, you want to start slowly circling the breasts before moving your massage towards the areola. There, you want to continue drawing circles in your massage. Avoid touching the nipples too quickly, you want to take your time and really activate all of the bodily senses and heighten your physical awareness.

As your body begins to really respond, you can start teasing the nipples. Alternate between light pinching, circles, and various touches to really stimulate the nerves in the nipples. Always take your time, touch slowly and intentionally, and pay attention to how your body is physically responding to the sensations that are being applied to it.

Once you have warmed your body up and have completed a thorough breast massage, you can work your way down to the yoni. Some people prefer to head down there quickly, whereas others like to draw their massage down slowly so that they can further enhance the experience. For the sake of pleasure and fulfillment, I recommend you take your time and work downwards slowly. Again, explore the various areas of your body between your breasts and your yoni and take some time to notice how differently they feel now that your body is activated and your senses are heightened.

Five Massage Techniques

Upon reaching your yoni, there are five primary massage techniques that are involved in a Tantric massage. These techniques will help you gain maximum benefit from your massage and will teach you how to activate various stimulations and sensations during sex.

You always want to mix up the methods you use, ideally using all five with each massage. You can alternate the tempo, variation, and order that you complete these techniques in to keep each massage effective and fulfilling for the recipient. Ideally, you don't want to allow your massages to become repetitive or predictable because this can take away from the overall experience of the massages.

When you are completing these massage methods, you should also take the time to simultaneously find ways to stimulate other areas on the body. This will help spread the orgasmic energy out to include all areas of the body, which will create an even more enjoyable experience from the massage. You might include the nipples, rub the thighs, massage the lower belly, or otherwise stimulate the body in alternative ways while also stimulating it through the yoni massage.

Circling

This method is simple and also happens to be one of the most commonly used ones when arousing a woman for sexual intercourse. For sexual intercourse, this method can often be used as a quick-fire opportunity to turn a woman on. During a Tantric massage you want to be slow and deliberate with your movements. Take your time, and work intentionally.

To complete the circling technique, you simply want to circle the tip of your finger around the clitoris. You should vary the size of your circles, as well as the pressure you are using on the clitoris. Alternate between various stimulations so that the area becomes highly aroused and activated and you are able to gain maximum pleasure from this area.

The clitoris itself and the surrounding area is considered to be one area on the female's body that has the highest amount of nerve endings. That is why many people rely on it for arousing a female. However, it is not the only area with a high number of nerve endings and should not be sought after as the only opportunity to arouse a woman. Make sure that you vacate this area after a while in order to stimulate other areas of the yoni.

Pushing and Pulling

The next method is a process of pushing and pulling the clitoris. This requires you to take your finger and slide it down the shaft of the clitoris. You want to do it on both sides, as some women are more sensitive in certain areas over others. Doing this will allow you to stimulate more of the clitoris, even more so than that which is generally stimulated by sexual intercourse or foreplay.

As you are doing this, take your time and alternate your pressures. Explore all areas of the shaft of the clitoris and notice what sensation is caused by each area. Feel each new energy as you touch various areas of the clitoris and apply various sensations on each area.

Tugging and Rolling

This process should be done gently, as each woman has a different threshold and doing this activity the wrong way can cause pain instead of pleasurable stimulation. On yourself, this is easy to gauge. However, if this is being done by someone else on you, be sure they are aware of what your threshold is. Use communication in order to ensure that they don't take it too far and take you out of the pleasure.

Tugging happens when you gently pull the clitoris away from the body, generally doing so using your index finger and your thumb. You want to do this by grasping the sides of the clitoris and tugging it back and forth. What that means is you can pull it out at different angles and even move it around while it is pulled out. You can also move around and tug at the sides of the lips of your vagina as well, as this often causes a highly pleasurable sensation for many women.

If you want to start rolling the clitoris, simply hold it firmly between your thumb and index finger and start rolling it around. It may feel as though you are making a tiny violin-movement with your fingers during this process. This is the part where many women like to increase the pressure, as it can stimulate the nerve endings in an entirely new way and draw someone closer to climax.

Tapping

This is as simple as it sounds: you simply want to use one or more fingers and begin tapping the clitoris in various rhythms. Ideally, you want to play around and see what your body responds to the most. You can even start tapping other areas of your yoni if you want to create a stimulation elsewhere, as well. Take your time, change up your rhythm, and use varying pressures in each tap to stimulate new sensations.

With this one, you always want to be careful not to overdo it. This is especially true if you are tapping someone else. Tapping can become painful if the pressure is too hard, and can become uncomfortable if the rhythm is too fast at the wrong time in the climax experience. Always be sure to pay close attention to signals from the body of the recipient to ensure that the experience is being well received and that you are not creating pain or taking away from the pleasure of the massage.

G-Spot Massage

The g-spot is a well-known area in the female yoni and yet many people are unaware as to where it is. Women and men alike often find this place to be allusive and struggle to discover it. As a woman giving a massage to yourself, it can be significantly easier to locate it. If you are getting a massage from someone else, they will know they have reached the g-spot when your pleasure heightens significantly.

In order to locate the g-spot, you want to insert two fingers into the vagina and curve them to make a c-shape. In behind the clitoris you will find a soft, spongy piece of skin. It often feels somewhat like a very soft bump in the vagina. This spot is filled with nerve endings and can create a significant amount of pleasure for a woman.

To properly massage the g-spot, you want to vary the speed of your strokes as well as the pressure. You can tickle the area, massage it, stroke it, or even tap it depending on what the massage recipient enjoys most. The more you play around, the more you will get an idea of what you like in this area and how it feels for you. If you want to maximize the pleasure of a g-spot massage, you can tickle the clitoris or place pressure directly above the pubic bone with your other hand. Both of these will increase the stimulation and make the experience even more enjoyable.

Edging

The goal when you are giving a Tantric massage is to almost orgasm over and over again. When you almost orgasm, this is called an "edge", or, "the edge of orgasm". Edging essentially means that you do this repeatedly by drawing yourself almost completely to a climax and then slowing down before it actually happens. This can take some practice as there reaches a point where if you simply slow down or stop the stimulation the orgasm will still happen but it will be significantly less enjoyable for the recipient. You need to learn to find where your edge is and play with it. As you become more experienced it will become a lot easier for you to find your edge, and it will also be a lot easier for you to physically draw out the orgasmic experience.

When you are cooling down between edges to prevent yourself from fully climaxing, you should place your hand over your heart. Take the time to feel your pulse, as this will keep your body grounded and connection and will help increase the emotional energy being experienced alongside the sexual energy. Once you have cooled down enough, you can start warming up again and bringing yourself back towards the edge.

You can choose how many edges you want to experience before you fully orgasm. However, it is important to note that your experience will be much more enjoyable if you edge multiple times before allowing yourself to orgasm. The more you edge, the more heightened your senses will be and therefore the more of an impact your orgasm will have on your entire body.

Tips When Giving a Yoni Massage to Yourself

When you give yourself a yoni massage, you want to take your time and be fluent about what you do. Even if you are capable of orgasming during your masturbation, approach this as a whole new experience. Discard everything you know about your own orgasms and your body, and use this as an opportunity to learn even more. If you come at this with an "all knowingness" there is a good chance that you will deny yourself pleasure because you only emphasize on certain areas or refuse to further explore your body.

Yoni massages require you to release your inhibitions, take some time to yourself and really enjoy the experience overall. You need to allow yourself to have a thorough and fulfilling experience in order for the massage to be successful. You do not want to have distractions or fear that someone is going to intrude on your experience and create a negative or traumatic effect around it. The yoni massage should always be a positive, pleasurable, and emotionally as well as physically fulfilling experience.

Tips When Giving a Yoni Massage to Someone Else

If you are giving a yoni massage to someone, there are some things you should first consider. If you have had intercourse with this person in the past, discard anything you know about their preferences. Aside from anything they strongly dislike, you should allow yourself to enter the situation with an open mind. Explore their body alongside them by massaging and using their physical and verbal communications as an opportunity to learn more about what they like and what they dislike.

Always be sure to pay close attention to verbal and non-verbal communications from the recipient. If your recipient begins to flinch excessively, it is likely that they are experiencing discomfort or potentially even pain. This can indicate excessive stimulation, and that is not a goal that you are trying to achieve. If they begin to flinch a lot or are shrinking under your touch too far, then slow down or remove the stimulation from that area and explore somewhere else for a while. Also, if they verbally tell you they do not like or do not want something, always respect their wishes. If you do not, you create a sense of distrust between yourself and the recipient and that can lead to a destruction of pleasure and can create troubles between yourself and the recipient. They should always feel as though they can trust you and as though your primary concern is their comfort and enjoyment. If you do not have consent to do something, do not do it. It is that simple.

Chapter 4
Tantric Massage for Men

Men and women vary greatly in their sexuality. Whereas women need a lot of foreplay and take much longer to climax, men are often turned on by a simple touch. Because of how easy it is for them to become turned on, they often skip over foreplay entirely and jump right into intercourse itself. Tantric massages can teach men to slow down and appreciate the experience of being touched. It also teaches them to have greater control over their climax which allows them to last longer during actual intercourse, as well as to have multiple orgasms during a single session of intercourse.

Giving a Tantric massage to a man is quite similar to giving one to a woman, although the erogenous zones will be quite a bit different since men are sexually different in physique compared to women. Of course, the sexual organs themselves are still important, but men tend to be turned on by different areas of the body, as well. Because of where these areas are located, this massage is best when done by someone else as it can be difficult for a man to reach them, let alone stimulate them.

How to Start

As with women, you want to start by warming the man up for the massage. The more prepared he is, the more sexually turned on he will be and therefore the more he will enjoy the experience. You really want to engage their entire body so that they can have a full-body orgasm. Most men are only familiar with ejaculation and the explosive feelings they get in their sexual areas when they are climaxing. Tantric massages can teach them to have full-bodied orgasms that allow them to experience the climax throughout the entire body instead of simply in the sexual region.

You want to start warming him up on his back. So, have the man lying on his stomach and get really comfortable in his position. Ideally, he should cross his hands under his head or above his head so that his back is nice and stretched out and open to the massage process. You want him to be really relaxed and open to the experience. Allow him to connect with his breath through relaxation and deep breathing.

Using a really nice massage oil, pour some onto the base of his spine and then work it in all the way up towards his shoulders. You should use your thumbs to work it in, always working next to the spine and never directly over it. Applying direct pressure to the spine during any type of massage can create discomfort and even injury in the delicate spinal discs. Always make sure that you are working in the muscle and tissue that runs along the spine. When working here, you want to be firm and intentional, but delicate and gentle. Too much pressure can create pain, so you want to make sure you are working with enough pressure to loosen the area without causing any level of discomfort.

Once you reach his shoulder blades, massage his entire upper back to relieve any tension he may be experiencing. You want to focus on the tops of the shoulders, the base of the neck as well as the neck itself, where the arm connects to the back, and under the shoulder blades. Use various pressures and rhythms to change it up and really draw him into a sense of relaxation and calmness. Make sure that the pressure you are using is always appropriate to the area to avoid discomfort or injury.

As he begins to completely relax and get into the "zone", start lightly tapping his back with the edges of your hands. You don't want to tap too hard, but you want it to be felt and noticeable. Tapping leads to a stimulation of sexual energy in males, and the nerve impulses that are triggered through this process will go straight to their genitals. Take your time and alternate between tapping and massaging for a few minutes as he gets more and more turned on.

Once your man becomes turned on by the experience, place a soft towel over his back and gently massage his back through the towel to absorb any excess oil or lotion that may be left over from the massage. Then, taking a deep breath, start running your lips up the base of his spine and all the way to the nape of his neck. When you are doing this, you want one lip to be gently brushing either side of his spine. Exhale slowly through the process to stimulate the nerves on his back. This will activate his sexual energies and draw them away from his genitals and up through his entire body, lending towards him being able to enjoy a full-bodied orgasm.

As you continue to get more sexual energy flowing through his body, use your hands and work up away from the base of his spine and up to his neck. Use your dominant hand and move slowly as you do it. You can rub it back and forth over a small section at a time or run it up and down the entire length of his back. Play around and see what works best, and change it up each time. This creates friction which generates heat and activates the nerves in his body even more. As you continue rubbing, pay attention to his shoulders before eventually working your way back down his body and to his butt.

Once you have completed these techniques, there is no doubt that your man's entire body will be aching for an orgasm. All of his nerves will be activated and stimulated and he will be more than ready for you to take him, or the other way around. However, there is still more massage left to go. The following section will describe the five best massage techniques to use on your man's sexual organs.

Five Massage Techniques

Now that he is warmed up, you can start working your hands towards his package. Remember, whenever you are massaging someone in such a sensitive area you want to be gentle and intentional. Never get rough, and never apply a significant amount of pressure as this can lead to intense pain and can destroy the entire process. You always want to be gentle and careful. Keep the communication open by listening to verbal and nonverbal cues as to whether or not your partner is enjoying the process. If at any point they get squirmy or start flinching a lot, it is likely that you are over stimulating them and you need to slow down or remove the stimulation from that area altogether until they can relax again.

Circling

When you are circling your man, it essentially means that you are working around the base of his shaft, where the penis connects to the body. You always want to be fairly intentional and apply a consistent amount of pressure here as it can be quite sensitive and if you are too soft it can tickle as opposed to feel satisfying. Take your time and explore the area, allowing your wrist and hand to touch his penis as a by-product of the circling massage.

Men have a very sensitive sexual zone and many are unaware of just how many nerve endings are present in their groin area. These areas are often overlooked during regular intercourse which leads to them never having been explored. You want to take your time, explore these areas, and help your man find out what feels good and what feels great. You can circle his package, or you can even rub your hands in small circles as you explore the area.

Rubbing

When men are masturbating or receiving a hand job the go-to action is to circle your fingers around the penis and start rubbing or grabbing your hand back-and-forth, stimulating sexual intercourse with the hand. While this can get the job done, it certainly doesn't allow for him to feel all of the pleasures of the area. When rubbing his shaft, don't close your fingers around his penis. Instead, keep your hand open and use two or three fingers to gently but intentionally rub around his penis.

The underside of the penis tends to be the most sensitive, particularly right underneath the head of the penis. You don't want to stay in this one area but bear in mind that this is where the most nerve endings are and this is where he is going to get the most pleasure from the experience. Think of it as your man's very own "g-spot".

If you want to add a little more pressure and change up the experience, you can cup the penis in your fingers and massage it using your thumb. This can make it easier to explore the underside of the shaft, apply friction, and make the massage more enjoyable for your man. Experiment with various pressures and positions to find out what kinds of rubbing he likes the most.

Pulling and Pushing

Again, this tends to be part of the "go-to" method for hand jobs or masturbating. It allows an intercourse-like stimulation to take place which can lead to ejaculation in a matter of minutes. However, it fails to allow for the entire area to be explored, let alone for all of his nerves to be activated. You want to take your time and gently tug and push various areas. Try pulling gently on his penis and then pushing your hand back down the shaft, without actually gripping any one area of the foreskin.

You can also use pulling and pushing on the testicles, though you want to be extremely gentle in this area. When pulling, never pull the testicles apart or pull them too hard or rigorously. Instead, simply cup both of them in your hand and very gently pull them until the skin appears to be slightly stretched out, and then press your cupped hand back towards his body. This very gentle and intentional movement can stimulate the nerves in his testicles, which are highly sensitive and extremely sexual. They have a major impact on his overall orgasm, and should certainly not be overlooked. However, you must always be very gentle and intentional in this area as they can be damaged or you can inflict pain extremely easily.

Tugging

With men, tugging of the penis can be highly sexual. Never tug on the testicles, however. This will cause pain or damage, or both.

Tugging the penis is easy, you simply want to grab it with a fair amount of pressure and start tugging it. Of course, you don't want to tug it like you're playing a game of tug-of-war. However, gently tugging it towards yourself can really begin to activate the sensations felt at the base of the shaft, where the penis connects to the body. It can also stimulate the area under your hand where friction is being created.

Never tug too hard, too long, or too many times in a row. Always keep this as an in-between movement to stimulate more nerves, without lingering on this move too long. Keeping it as a surprise now-and-again type movement can ensure that it remains pleasurable for as long as you use it with your man.

Tickling

The tickling of the penis and sexual area can be highly enjoyable for your man. You never want to tickle to the point of making it uncomfortable, but fairly firm tickling motions around the penis and testicle area can heighten the enjoyment he feels from the experience. It allows you to activate even more nerve endings with an entirely new sensation outside of rubbing and tugging.

When you are tickling, you want to act as though you are actually tickling him but apply a little more pressure than you would if you were intending to tickle someone to make them laugh. If you tickle him to the point of making him laugh, you will break the pleasure and create discomfort because he will be over stimulated. You want to find a happy medium where you can create a new sensation and stimulate him in a new way without taking him out of the pleasure.

Edging

Edging is an important part of Tantric massage because it helps create an increase in anticipation which maximizes the pleasure felt from the massage, as well as from the orgasm or orgasms that follow. You always want to make sure that you are paying attention to your partner's cues to ensure that you slow down and prevent them from climaxing too soon, as the longer the experience is the more enjoyable it will be and the more powerful the orgasm will be.

Men are often known to climax much faster than a woman, with an average of 4-8 minutes from initial stimulation to complete ejaculation. Depending on your partner, this may be shorter or longer, either of which is completely okay. You want to get to know your partner enough that you can tell when they are nearing climax and then you can slow down, stop, or change the stimulation to prevent them from climaxing until you intend for them too. It can take some time to find when the exact moment is that they can come back down from the edge and when it has gotten to the point where even stopping stimulation won't change the course of the orgasm. If you don't stop in time the first few times, that is completely normal. The more you get to know your partner on this intimate level the easier it will be. Additionally, the more they get used to the experience of Tantric massage the easier it will be to have control over their climax and hold it back so that they last longer.

One of the benefits of Tantric massage for men is that it teaches them to edge longer and prevent themselves from climaxing too quickly. This means that they can last longer, which heightens the enjoyment for themselves as their orgasm will be much more powerful. It also means that their female partner will be more likely to reach orgasm during their sexual intercourse because he can last the 20 minutes or so that is needed for a female to orgasm during sex.

Tips for Giving a Tantric Massage to a Man

When you are giving a tantric massage you always want to be very open and receptive to the recipient. You should be aware of what their nonverbal and verbal cues are so that you are prepared to change the course of the experience to suit their needs and make it enjoyable for them.

Always make sure that you are listening to their communications, otherwise, you may break the trust and intimacy between you and your partner. Trust and intimacy in the moment are a large part of what makes the experience so enjoyable, as they help the recipient open up to the experience and relax completely. Your partner should always consent to the experience and they should always feel comfortable and calm during the process. You want Tantric massages to be a positive and pleasant experience for the recipient so that they can enjoy all of the benefits that Tantric massages have to offer.

Chapter 5
Enhancing the Experience

There are many ways to enhance the experience that both sexes have when they enjoy a Tantric massage. These come from emotional enhancements to physical enhancements, and they can greatly increase the benefit of the massage as well as the experience overall. If you want to further increase the pleasure and benefits that you or your partner gains from a Tantric massage, try the follow techniques and tricks.

Trust and Intimacy

As you learned in the previous two chapters, trust and intimacy are very important when you are giving a Tantric massage. It allows the recipient to feel comfortable in their vulnerability and truly enjoy the massage to the full extent. They are able to trust that their partner will be caring towards them and their desires and that the experience will be pleasurable and positive.

Trust and intimacy can be built in many ways. Outside of the massage, you can build it by genuinely listening to your partner and addressing their needs and concerns. It can be built by earning your partner's respect and trust and creating intimate moments with them such as through planning fun dates or experiences together, or even simply holding their hand and kissing them more. Even though these don't directly correlate with the massage itself, they can have a major impact on the level of trust and intimacy felt between partners so that it is already present before the massage even takes place. If you are a female and you are working on massaging yourself, you can also work in building up your trust and intimacy with yourself by trusting your intuition and doing what feels positive to you.

Within the massage, trust and intimacy can be built through movement and communication. It is not likely that much verbal communication will be used during the massage, so it is important that both partners learn to really understand each other's non-verbal communication patterns. As you have already learned, excessive squirming or flinching generally means too much stimulation is being applied and they are becoming uncomfortable. By noticing this, you can slow down or move the stimulation elsewhere for a few moments to help alleviate the discomfort and bring them back into pleasure. The more you get to know how your partner physically communicates, the sooner you can reduce these discomforts and keep the experience positive overall.

The same goes in the opposite direction as well. If your partner appears to lack any level of response to the experience, it is either because they are not feeling open to the experience or they are not being stimulated enough by the touching. You either need to help them relax further or use a little more pressure or change up the rhythm with your touching.

As you get to know your partner more in this new way, it will become a lot easier for you to stimulate their entire body and bring them towards phenomenal orgasmic experiences. Still, the body can feel different on different days, so you always want to be open and aware of the communications that are being shared with your partner so that you can keep the massage positive and pleasurable.

Engage the Senses

One of the reasons why Tantric massages are so beneficial in creating a full-body experience is because they incorporate the full body into the orgasm. This is primarily done through the massaging process, but it can be done through many other methods as well. The more senses you incorporate into the massage, the more the experience is going to be enjoyed by both the person giving the massage and the person receiving it.

The primary senses that can be included in a Tantric massage are smell, hearing, touching, and seeing. Smell is an important one as it can stimulate a positive experience overall. If the smell is unpleasant in the area, the person may never fully relax or enjoy the massage. Although music will likely fall into the background, it can really amp up the experience by eliminating excessively quiet and potentially awkward background sounds. Touching is obviously stimulated by the massage but can be stimulated in other ways as well. And finally, sight can be stimulated through the massage as well. The best massage will incorporate each one of these into the experience.

Scented Candles

Having scented candles or wax melts on in the room is a great way to create a romantic and calming sense of smell. Some smells, such as lavender, rose, geranium, and clary sage have been proven to help eliminate stress and increase the amount of peace a person feels mentally. This can help create a calmer atmosphere and bring the massage giver and receiver both into a more present and relaxed state. If you are using candles, always be sure that they are placed somewhere safe and that they won't catch anything on fire or get knocked over in the process.

Scented Massage Oil

Scented massage oils or lotions are another great way to incorporate smells into the massage. If you have any other scents present, such as scented candles, always make sure that you are choosing two smells that will complement each other. The massage giver can take the process a step further by applying the scented lotion to their own body before giving the massage, as this can create a more positive aroma from themselves as well, especially as the heat of their own body diffuses the smell around them. Avoid wearing perfumes or anything strong during this process as it can be unpleasant for the recipient, particularly if they are in close quarters with you, which they will be.

Low Lighting

As with anything romantic, low lighting is a great way to calm the sense of sight and bring a more relaxed state to the atmosphere. You can simply put on a small lamp and turn off the main light, or apply translucent drapes to a naturally lit window to dim the light in the room.

If you want to add an even more romantic or calming tone to space, you can turn out all of the lights and turn on one or two Himalayan salt lamps. Because of their design, they create an ambient lighting that is rose pink in color, which can create a highly romantic and serene environment for the massage to be given in. How you choose to dim the lights is up to you, but it is highly encouraged and recommended that you ditch harsh overhead lighting and go with something more comfortable and soothing.

Sight Stimulation

Giving a Tantric massage in a room that is excessively messy or filled with clutter can take away from the experience. You may find yourself tripping over clutter, or you may find that it's simply hard to relax with everything around you. Even if you close your eyes, it can still be hard to tune out all of the chaos that surrounds you at the moment. Before you begin giving or receiving a Tantric massage, take some time to completely clean your environment. This will keep everything clean and clutter free, helping you to completely calm yourself and relax your mind. The more relaxed you are, the more open and receptive you will be to the experience and therefore the more pleasurable the Tantric massage will be for both the giver and the receiver.

Another thing you can pay attention to is the clothes you are wearing. As the person giving the massage, wearing anything excessive or too vibrant can actually detract from the quality of the massage. You want to wear something simple, relaxing, and void of loud or clashing colors or patterns. Or, if you're close enough with your partner, stick to your underwear or even nothing at all.

Soft Music

Soft music is a great way to enhance the experience. You can go for strictly instrumental tones like piano melodies or classical music, or you can go for one that has a low and soft voice that lulls you into a peaceful state of relaxation. The only goal is to ensure that the music does not become too fast-paced, loud, or filled with harsh or sharp voices or tones. The music should be calming, relaxing, and soothing. Music is excellent for filling in the background noise to keep the overall experience comforting. Without it, some people may become distracted by background sounds. Others may prefer complete silence. Simply communicate with your partner to find their preference.

If you do choose to put on music, one good idea is to make sure that you choose a playlist that is long enough to last the entire massage. You don't want to have to get up throughout the massage to change the song or put the music back on because it has turned off again or the album has ended.

Incorporate Other Objects

Although the touching senses are going to be primarily activated through the physical massage itself, it can also be enhanced through other methods. During the massage you can wear gloves such as fleece or leather ones to gain a new sensation, or you can incorporate feathers, silk, pearls, or even soft faux fur materials to create new sensations. You can also wear clothes that are silky or soft so that when your body touches your partners they are greeted with pleasant materials that feel nice against the skin. In addition to these methods, you should also choose a comfortable surface with comfortable bedding, blankets, or other materials underneath the recipient. Silk, satin, fleece, faux fur, and other materials can be used underneath. Ask the recipient what their favorite is, as some dislike certain textures or prefer others.

There are many other ways that you can increase the joy experienced from the massage, as well. Simply communicate with your partner and learn more about what they liked and what they dislike, and things they might be open to or want to try during the massage. The more you learn about your partner and their preferences and dislikes, the more you can creatively explore the world of Tantric massages and further enhance the experience for both partners involved.

Conclusion

Tantric massage is a sensual, sexual massage that incorporates the entire body to stimulate sexual energy. While most people think it is purely a sexual act, they are in fact wrong. Tantric massages are sexual in energy, but they are primarily focused on creating an overall sense of pleasure for the recipient. They can have many benefits, including an enhanced overall sense of self-esteem and confidence, enhanced pleasure, greater joy from sexual intercourse, and relief from sexual traumas or other types of abuse. True Tantric massages are not intended to end in sexual intercourse, but rather in the recipient having an orgasm as a result of the massage itself.

As a female, you can give yourself a tantric massage or you can receive one from someone else. As a male, it is much easier if you receive one from someone else. Tantric massages can be received from a professional massage therapist who is trained in Tantra, or they can be learned and given between partners. It is important that you choose to get the massage from someone who you are comfortable with and who you trust.

I hope this book was able to teach you about Tantric massage and the many benefits it has to offer. If you want to further explore the world of Tantric massages, you should work together with your partner or a professional to learn more. This way, you can explore your own sexual energies and potentially the energies of someone else, too.

The next step is to find yourself a Tantric massage partner and begin practicing. Take your time and give yourself the opportunity to make mistakes, because you won't master everything the first time around. Learning to edge your partner can take some practice, but eventually, you will master it and it will be simple for you to accomplish.

Lastly, I ask that you please take the time to rate this book on Amazon. Your honest feedback would be greatly appreciated.

Thank you.

Book Description

Tantric massage is wonderful massage therapy that stimulates sexual energies to have a variety of outcomes. Many people falsely believe that Tantric massages are a sexual act, likely because of the way they use sexual energy to stimulate pleasure in the recipient. The reality is that a true Tantric massage will not end in a sexual act and will instead end in the recipient experiencing a full-body orgasm as a result of the pleasurable massage they receive.

Giving a Tantric massage is a lot easier than it may seem. However, there are some strategies and techniques that you need to know before you get started. *"Tantric Massage*: The Ultimate Beginners Guide to Tantric Massage Techniques" will teach you exactly what you should know before you start practicing Tantric massages on someone else.

You will learn about:

- What the massage is, exactly

- Why it is beneficial for men

- Why it is beneficial for women

- How to give a Tantric massage to both men and women

- Things to consider

- Tips to enhance the process

If you are ready to begin exploring the world of Tantric massages and the benefits they can have, this book is the perfect place for you to get started.